Easy Low-Carb Recipe

The Keto Diet Cookbook for Weight Loss and Improve Your Metabolism

Aida Harris

Copyright © 2021 Aida Harris

All rights reserved.

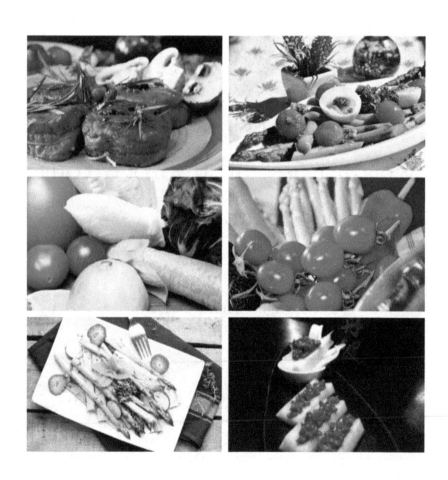

Table of content

4

Low-Carb Menu Planning and One-Dish Meals

In the vast majority of the dishes in this book, the biggest source of carbohydrates is vegetables. I trust we can agree that this is the healthiest possible source of carbohydrates, no? Vegetables, however, are more than that— they are the most flavorful source of carbohydrates in our diet, and by cooking our very low-carb proteins with a variety of vegetables, we can create a widely varied, delicious, exciting low-carb cuisine. However, this will sometimes mean that your carbohydrate allowance for a given meal is completely used up by the vegetables in your soup or skillet supper. This, then, becomes a classic one-dish meal, and a beautiful thing it is.

What about My Carb-Eating Family?

No reason not to serve a carbohydrate food on the side, if your family will be bereft without it. However, I must say that many of the quickest, easiest carbohydrate side dishes—instant mashed potatoes, quick-cooking rice, whack- em-on-the-counter biscuits and rolls—are just as processed and nutrient-

depleted as they can be and are also among the carbohydrates with the highest, most devastating blood sugar impact. Better to serve whole-wheat pita bread; corn or whole-wheat tortillas; one of the less damaging pastas (Jerusalem artichoke pasta, widely available at health food stores, has a relatively modest blood sugar impact and tastes like "regular" pasta); or potatoes you've cut into wedges, sprinkled with olive oil, and roasted in your toaster oven for about 15 minutes at

400°F (200°C, gas mark 6). If your family loves rice, well, brown rice is *hugely* superior to white rice, let alone Minute Rice, but it's nobody's idea of a 15-minute food. However, it reheats beautifully in the microwave. You could make a good-size pot of it over the weekend, stash it in the refrigerator, and use it later in the week. When you need it, just spoon out however much your family will need for the meal at hand, put it in a covered microwaveable container with a tablespoon (15 ml) or so of water, and nuke it on 70 percent power for a few minutes.

Anyway, the point is that if your family simply *insists* on a concentrated carbohydrate, serve it on the side. And because you love them, make it one of the less processed, less damaging carbohydrates.

What's a "Serving"?

I've gotten a couple of queries from folks who bought *500 Low-Carb Recipes* and want to know how big a serving size is, so I thought I'd better address the matter.

To be quite honest, folks, there's no great technical determination going on here. For the most part, a "serving" is based on what I think would make a reasonable portion, depending on the carbohydrate count, how rich the dish is, and for main dishes, the protein count. You just divide the dish up into however many portions the recipe says, and you can figure the carb counts on the recipes are accurate. In some cases I've given you a range—"3 or 4 servings," or whatever. In those cases, I've told you how many servings the carb counts are based on, and you can do a little quick mental estimating if, say, you're serving 4 people when I've given the count for 3.

Of course, this "serving" thing is flukey. People are different sizes and have different appetites. For all I know, you have three children under 5 who might reasonably split one adult-size portion. On the other hand, you might have one 17-year-old boy who's shot up from 5'5" to 6'3" in the past year, and what looks like 4 servings to me will be a quick snack for him. You'll just have to eyeball what fraction of the whole dish you're eating and go from there.

I've had a few people tell me they'd rather have specific serving sizes—like

"1 cup" or the like. I see a few problems with this. First of all, it sure won't work with things like steak or chops —I'd have to use weights, instead, and then all my readers would have to run out and buy scales. Secondly, my recipes generally call for things like, "1/2 head cauliflower" or "2 stalks celery." These things vary in size a bit, and as a result yield will fluctuate a bit, too. Also, if one of my recipes calls for "1 1/2 pounds (680 g) boneless, skinless chicken breasts" and your package is labeled "1.65 pounds (750 g)," I don't expect you to whack off the difference to get the portions exact.

In short, I hate to have to weigh and measure everything, and I'm betting that a majority of my readers feel the same way, even if some do not. So I apologize to those who like exact measures, but this is how it's going to be for now, at any rate.

What's With the Info about Stuff other than Carbs and Protein?

You'll notice that in places in this book I've included notes regarding other nutritional components of some of the recipes. Most notably, I've included the calorie count if it seems quite low and the calcium or potassium count if it seems quite high. The reason for this is simple: Many people are trying to watch their calories as well as their carbs, and calling their attention to those dishes in this book that are particularly low in calories seemed helpful. Likewise, my e- mail tells me that the two nutrients low-carbers are most concerned they're *not* getting are calcium and potassium. So letting you know when a recipe is a good source of these nutrients also seemed helpful.

All of the recipes do, of course, include the carbohydrate, fiber, usable carbs, and protein counts.

On the Importance of Reading Labels

Do yourself a favor and get in the habit of reading the label on every food product, and I do mean every food product, that has one. I have learned from long, hard, repetitive experience that food processors can, will, and do put sugar, corn syrup, corn starch, and other nutritionally empty, carb-filled garbage into every conceivable food product. You will shave untold thousands of grams of carbohydrates off your intake over the course of a year by simply looking for the product that has *no added junk*.

There are also a good many classes of food products out there to which sugar is virtually always added — the cured meats immediately come to mind. There is almost

10

always sugar in sausage, ham, bacon, hot dogs, liverwurst, and the like. You will look in vain for sugarless varieties of these products. However, you will

find that there is quite a range of carb counts because some manufacturers add more sugar than others. I have seen ham that has 1 gram of carbohydrates per serving, and I have seen ham that has 6 grams of carbohydrates per serving— that's a 600 percent difference! Likewise, I've seen hot dogs that have 1 gram of carbohydrates apiece, and I've seen hot dogs that have 5 grams of carbohydrates apiece.

If you're in a position where you can't read the labels—for instance, at the deli counter at the grocery store—then ask questions. The nice deli folks will be glad to read the labels on the ham and salami for you, and they can tell you what goes into the various items they make themselves. You'll want to ask at the meat counter, too, if you're buying something they've mixed up themselves—Italian sausage, marinated meats, or whatever. I have found that if I state simply that I have a medical condition that requires that I be very careful about my diet—and I don't show up at the busiest hour of the week!—folks are generally very nice about this sort of thing.

In short, become a food sleuth. After all, you're paying your hard-earned money for this stuff, and it is quite literally going to become a part of you. Pay at least as much attention to your food shopping as you would if you were buying a car or a computer!

Appliances for 15-Minute Meals

There are a few kitchen appliances that you'll use over and over to make the recipes in this book. They're all quite common, and I feel safe in assuming that the majority of you have most, if not all, of these appliances.

A microwave oven. Surely everybody is clear by now on how quickly these both thaw and cook all sorts of things. We'll use your microwave over and over again to cook one part of a dish while another part is on the stove—to heat a broth, steam a vegetable, or cook the bacon that we're going to use as a topping.

It is assumed in these recipes that you have a microwave oven with a turntable; most of them have been made this way for quite a while now. If your microwave doesn't have a turntable, you'll have to interrupt whatever else you're doing and turn your food a few times during its microwaving time to avoid uneven cooking.

Also, be aware that microwaves vary in power, and my suggestions for power settings and times are therefore approximate. You'll learn pretty quickly whether your microwave is about the same power as mine or stronger or weaker.

One quick note about thawing things in the microwave: If you're coming home and pulling something right out of the freezer, you'll probably use the

microwave to thaw it, and that's fine. However, if you can think of what you'd like to eat ahead of time, you can thaw in the fridge or even on the counter. (Wrap things in several layers of old newspaper if you're going to be gone for many hours and the day is warm.

This will help keep things from going beyond thawing to spoiling.)

A good compromise is to thaw things most of the way in the microwave and then let them finish at room temperature. You retain more juices this way, but sometimes there's just no time for this.

A blender. You'll use this, or a stick blender, once in a while to puree something. You could probably use a food processor, instead. For that matter, while I use a standard-issue blender with a jar, there's no reason not to use one of those hand-held blenders.

A food processor. Chopping, grinding, and shredding ingredients by hand just doesn't fit into our time frame in many cases. If you don't yet own a food processor, a simple one that has an S-blade, plus a single disc that slices on one side and shreds on the other, shouldn't set you back more than $50 to $75.

An electric tabletop grill. Made popular by former Heavyweight Champion George Foreman, these appliances are everywhere. Mr. Foreman's version is quite good, but you can buy a cheaper version for all of 20 bucks. The burger chapter of this book assumes you have one of these appliances, but you can cook your burgers in a skillet instead or in some cases under the broiler. However, since these methods don't cook from both sides at once, you'll spend a few more minutes cooking this way than you would with the grill.

A slow cooker. What, I hear you cry, is a slow cooker doing in a book of *fast* recipes? Answering reader demand, that's what! I've gotten bunches of requests for slow cooker recipes from readers. Obviously, none of the slow cooker recipes will be done in 15 minutes. Instead, they require 15 minutes or less *prep time*, and that's including both the time to assemble the ingredients in the pot and the time to finish the dish and get it on the table when you get home.

If you don't have a slow cooker, consider picking one up. They're not expensive, and I see perfectly good ones all the time at thrift shops and yard sales for next to nothing. Keep your eyes open.

Bacon Blue Cheese Omelet

Here are three of my favorite things—wrapped in eggs, another of my favorite things!

> 3 slices bacon
> 1/4 Granny Smith or other crisp, tart apple, thinly sliced
> 2 teaspoons butter, divided
> 2 eggs, beaten
> 1 ounce (28 g) crumbled blue cheese

Start the bacon cooking in the microwave—if you don't own a microwave bacon rack, a glass pie plate will work just fine. (In my microwave, 3 to 4 minutes on High is about right, but microwave power varies.) While the bacon's cooking, melt 1 teaspoon of butter in your omelet pan over medium- high heat. Add the apples and fry for 2 to 3 minutes per side or until they're slightly golden. Remove the apple slices and keep them on hand.

Melt the remaining butter in the skillet, slosh it about, and make your omelet according to *Dana's Easy Omelet Method*, using nonstick cooking spray if necessary. Arrange the fried apples on half the omelet, top with the blue cheese, cover the pan, and turn the burner to low.

Go check on that bacon! If it needs another minute, do that now, while the cheese is melting. Then drain it and crumble it over the now-melted blue cheese. Fold and serve.

Yield: 1 serving, with 6 grams of carbohydrates and 1 gram of fiber, for a total of 5 grams of usable carbs and 23 grams of protein.

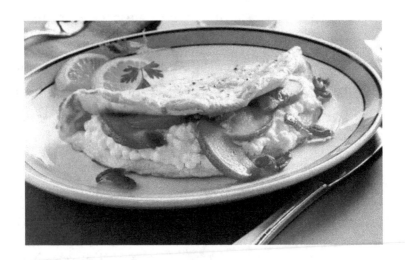

Cheese and Pear Omelets

I never played around with chive cream cheese before working on the new recipes for this book. What a versatile ingredient it is! This omelet is a wonderful, unusual combination of flavors.

  1/4 pear
  1 tablespoon (14 g) butter
  2 eggs
  3 tablespoons (38 g) whipped cream cheese
    with chives

Slice your pear quarter quite thin. Melt the butter in your omelet pan and

sauté the pear slices until they've soften a little more. Fork them out onto a plate and reserve.

Scramble up your eggs and pour them into the omelet pan. Cook as described in *Dana's Easy Omelet method*. When the liquid egg has stopped running, turn the burner to low and spoon in the chive cream cheese in little bits, distributing it over half the egg. Top with the pear slices, cover, and cook until the cheese is melted. Fold, plate, and devour!

Yield: 1 serving, with 362 calories, 31 grams fat, 13 grams protein, 9 grams carbohydrate, 1 gram dietary fiber, and 8 grams usable carb.

Chili Lime Pork Omelet

This is one of those omelets that makes it clear that eggs ain't just for breakfast anymore—this is definitely hearty enough for dinner. The *Chili Lime Pork* is very quick to make and keeps well in a closed container in the fridge.

2 eggs, beaten
1 to 2 teaspoons oil
1/4 batch *Chili Lime Pork Strips*
1/4 avocado, sliced
1/4 cup (29 g) shredded Monterey Jack cheese
Sour cream
Salsa

Make your omelet according to *Dana's Easy Omelet Method*. Arrange the *Chili Lime Pork* strips on half the omelet and top with the avocado and the cheese. Cover, turn the burner to low, and let it cook for a minute or two to melt the cheese and finish setting the eggs. Fold and serve. Top with sour cream, salsa, or both if desired.

Yield: 1 serving, with 6 grams of carbohydrates and 2 grams of fiber, for a total of 4 grams of usable carbs and 42 grams of protein

"Clean the Fridge" Omelet

The name is not a joke—I made this omelet up out of whatever I found kicking around in the refrigerator, needing to be used up before it went bad. The results were definitely good enough to make it again.

> 1/2 red bell pepper, cut into thin strips
> 1/4 medium onion, thinly sliced
> 3 tablespoons (45 ml) olive oil
> 2 eggs, beaten
> 1 ounce (28 g) jalapeño jack cheese, shredded or sliced
> 1/2 avocado, sliced

In your skillet over medium-high heat, sauté the pepper and onion in the oil until the onion is translucent and the pepper is going limp. Remove from the pan and keep on hand. If your pan isn't nonstick, give it a shot of nonstick cooking spray before putting it back on the burner and increasing the heat a touch to high. Make your omelet according to *Dana's Easy Omelet Method*. Put the cheese on half the omelet and top with the avocado, then the pepper and onion. Cover, turn the burner to low, and let it cook until the cheese is melted. Fold and serve.

Yield: 1 serving, with 14 grams of carbohydrates and 6 grams of fiber, for a total of 8 grams of usable carbs and 21 grams of protein.

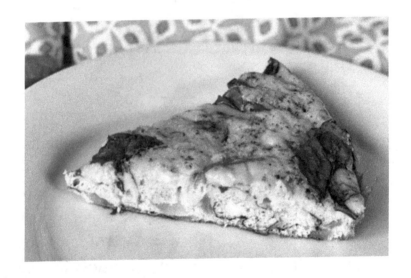

Curried Cheese and Olive Omelets

This was originally a spread for English muffins and the like, but it makes a wicked omelet. I know that this combination of ingredients sounds a little odd, but the flavor is magical.

> 1 cup (115 g) shredded cheddar cheese
> 5 or 6 scallions, finely sliced, including the crisp part of the green
> I can (4.25 ounces, or 120 g) chopped ripe olives, drained
> 3 tablespoons (42 g) mayonnaise
> 1/2 teaspoon curry powder
> 6 eggs, beaten

Simply plunk the cheese, scallions, olives, mayonnaise, and curry powder in a mixing bowl and combine well. Now, make omelets according to *Dana's*

Easy Omelet Method, using the cheese-and-olive mixture as the filling. As the 6 eggs suggests, this makes 3 omelets. If there's only one of you, however, just use 2 eggs. The cheese mixture will keep well for a couple of days in a closed container in the refrigerator, letting you make fabulous omelets in far less than 15 minutes for a few days running.

Tomato-Mozzarella Omelet

Sliced tomatoes and mozzarella are a time-honored Italian appetizer—and they make a great omelet filling, too.

2 eggs, beaten
1/3 cup (38 g) shredded mozzarella cheese
1/2 small tomato, sliced
2 tablespoons (6 g) chopped fresh basil

Make your omelet according to *Dana's Easy Omelet Method*. Cover half the omelet with the cheese and then top with the tomato slices. Cover, turn the burner to low, and let it cook for 2 to 3 minutes or until the cheese is melted. Scatter the basil over the filling, fold, and serve.

Yield: 1 serving, with 5 grams of carbohydrates and 1 gram of fiber, for a total of 4 grams of usable carbs and 20 grams of protein.

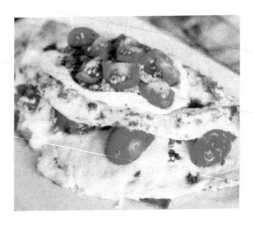

Kasseri Tapenade Omelet

This is full of cool Greek flavors! Look for jars of tapenade, an olive relish, in big grocery stores. Kasseri is a Greek cheese; all my local grocery stores carry it, so I'm guessing yours do, too.

 2 to 3 teaspoons (10 to 15 ml) olive oil
 2 eggs, beaten
 1 ounce (28 g) kasseri cheese, sliced or
 shredded 1 1/2 tablespoons (12 g) tapenade

Cover half the omelet with the cheese and then top with the tapenade. Cover, turn the burner to low, and let it cook for a couple of minutes until the cheese is melted. Fold and serve.

Yield: 1 serving, with 4 grams of carbohydrates, no fiber, and 18 grams of protein.

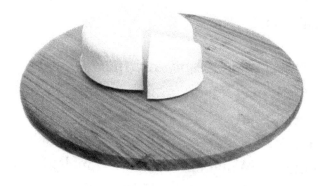

Smoked Salmon and Goat Cheese Scramble

Sounds fancy, I know, but this takes almost no time and is very impressive. It's terrific to make for a special brunch or a late-night supper. A simple green salad with a classic vinaigrette dressing would be perfect with this.

4 eggs1/2 cup (120 ml) heavy cream
1 teaspoon dried dill weed
4 scallions
1/4 pound (115 g) chevre (goat cheese)
1/4 pound (115 g) moist smoked salmon
1 to 2 tablespoons (14 to 28 g) butter

Whisk the eggs together with the cream and dill weed. Slice the scallions thin, including the crisp part of the green. Cut the chèvre—it will have a texture similar to cream cheese—into little hunks. Coarsely crumble the smoked

salmon.

In a big (preferably nonstick) skillet, melt the butter over medium-high heat. (If your skillet doesn't have a nonstick surface, give it a shot of nonstick cooking spray before adding the butter.) When the butter's melted, add the scallions first and sauté them for just a minute.

Add the eggs and cook, stirring frequently, until they're halfway set—about 1 minute to 90 seconds. Add the chèvre and smoked salmon, continue cooking and stirring until the eggs are set, and serve.

Yield: 3 servings, each with 5 grams of carbohydrates and 1 gram of fiber, for a total of 4 grams of usable carbs and 27 grams of protein.

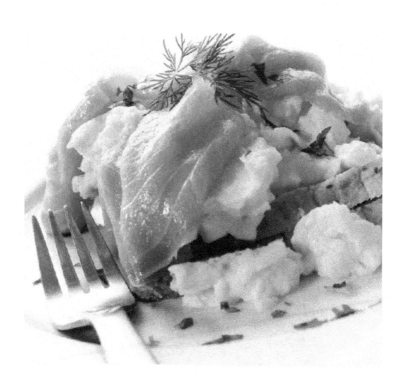

Deviled Ham and Eggs

If you don't have leftover ham lying around the house, you can buy modest-size chunks of pre-cooked ham in any grocery store. It's useful stuff!

> 1/2 tablespoon butter
> 1/2 cup (75 g) smallish ham cubes
> 1/4 cup (40 g) chopped onion
> 3 eggs
> 1 teaspoon spicy brown or Dijon mustard
> 1 teaspoon prepared horseradish

Melt the butter in a small skillet over medium heat. Add the ham and onion and sauté until the onion is translucent and the ham has a touch of gold. Scramble the eggs with the mustard and horseradish and pour them over the ham and onion in the skillet. Scramble until the eggs are set and serve.

Yield: 1 serving, with 8 grams of carbohydrates (less if you use really low- carb ham) and 1 gram of fiber, for a total of 7 grams of usable carbs and 29 grams of protein.

Parmesan Rosemary Eggs

This is so simple and so wonderful. If you like Italian food, you have to try this. It's also easy to double or triple.

> 3 eggs
> 2 tablespoons (28 ml) heavy cream
> 1/4 cup (25 g) grated Parmesan cheese
> 1/2 teaspoon ground rosemary
> 1/2 teaspoon minced garlic
> 1/2 tablespoon butter

* You can use whole, dried rosemary, but you'll have little needles in your food. If you do use whole rosemary, increase the amount to 1 teaspoon.

Whisk together the eggs, cream, cheese, rosemary, and garlic. Put a medium- size skillet over medium-high heat (if it isn't nonstick, give it a shot of nonstick cooking spray first). When the pan is hot, add the butter, give the egg mixture one last stir to make sure the cheese hasn't settled to the bottom, and then pour the egg mixture into the skillet. Scramble until the eggs are set and serve.

Yield: 1 serving, with 3 grams of carbohydrates, a trace of fiber, and 25 grams of protein.

Moroccan Scramble

With all these vegetables, this is a meal in itself. It's exotic and fabulous.

1 tablespoon 15 ml. olive oil
1/4 cui 40 g chopped onion
1/2 teaspoon minced garlic or 1 clove garlic, crushed
1 tablespoon (8 g) tapenade
1/4 cup (45 g) canned diced tomatoes
3 eggs
1/2 teaspoon ground cumin
2 tablespoons (2 g) chopped fresh cilantro
Salt and pepper

In a skillet, heat the olive oil over high heat and start sautéing the onion and garlic. When the onion is translucent, add the tapenade and tomatoes and stir. Now, whisk the eggs with the cumin and pour the eggs into the vegetable mixture. Scramble until mostly set and then add the cilantro and scramble until done. Salt and pepper to taste and serve.

Yield: 1 serving, with 11 grams of carbohydrates and 1 gram of fiber, for a total of 10 grams of usable carbs and 18 grams of protein.

French Country Scramble

This is for anyone who doesn't think that eggs can be elegant.

> 1/2 cup (60 g) shredded Gruyère cheese
> 4 ounces (115 g) sliced mushrooms
> 6 eggs
> 2 canned artichoke hearts, chopped
> 1 tablespoon (14 g) butter
> 3 scallions, coarsely sliced

If you haven't purchased your mushrooms already sliced, slice then up while you slice the scallions. In a large, heavy skillet over medium-high heat, sauté the mushrooms and scallions in the butter. When the mushrooms have turned darker, add the artichoke hearts (I just slice mine right into the skillet) and stir the whole thing up. Then beat the eggs, add them to the skillet, and scramble the whole thing. When the eggs are about half-set, add the cheese and scramble until done. Serve.

Hangtown Fry

This is a very famous dish originating, I believe, in the Gold Rush days of California.

8 large oysters

2 tablespoons (16 g) low-carb bake mix or 2 tablespoons (20 g) rice protein powder

4 tablespoons (55 g) butter

4 eggs

2 tablespoons (28 ml) cream

2 tablespoons (10 g) grated Parmesan cheese

2 tablespoons (8 g) chopped fresh parsley

Coat the oysters with the bake mix or protein powder, either by putting the bake mix or protein powder in a shallow dish and rolling the oysters in it or by shaking them in a small brown paper bag with the mix in it.

Melt the butter over medium heat in a large, heavy skillet. Add the oysters and fry until golden all over, about 5 to 7 minutes.

While the oysters are frying, beat the eggs and the cream together. When the oysters are golden, pour the beaten eggs into the skillet and scramble until set. Divide between 2 serving plates, sprinkle a tablespoon (5 g) of Parmesan and a tablespoon (4 g) of parsley over each portion, and serve.

Yield: 2 servings, each with 5 grams of carbohydrates and 1 gram of fiber, for a total of 4 grams of usable carbs and 21 grams of protein.

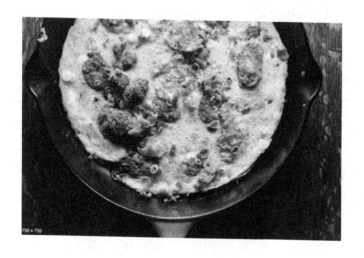

Cottage Egg Scramble

Eggs scrambled with cottage cheese are surprisingly good, and of course the cottage cheese adds nutrients the eggs lack—most notably calcium. With a salad on the side, this is a great simple supper for a tired night.

4 eggs
1/2 cup (115 g) small-curd cottage cheese
1/8 teaspoon dried basil
1/2 green pepper, finely chopped
1 tablespoon butter
1/4 cup (29 g) shredded cheddar cheese

Beat the eggs and cottage cheese together and stir in the basil. In a large, heavy skillet over medium-high heat, sauté the green pepper in the butter (you might want to give that skillet a shot of nonstick cooking spray first). When the pepper is getting a little soft, add the egg mixture and scramble. When the eggs are almost set, add the cheddar and continue scrambling until the eggs are completely set. Serve.

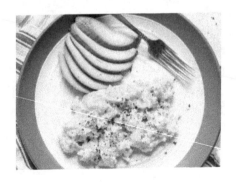

15-Minute Tortilla Tricks

Yes, there are low-carbohydrate tortillas! They're made by La Tortilla Factory, and they're loaded with fiber, which is why they're low carb—each tortilla has 12 grams of carbohydrate and 9 grams of fiber, for a total of just 3 grams of usable carbs.

As the popularity of low-carb dieting has increased, these low-carb tortillas have become easier to find in stores—I know a couple of places that carry them here in Bloomington, Indiana, and it's not like we're the retail capital of the universe. Look around. If you can't find them, consider asking a local health food store to special order them for you—most health food stores are really helpful about special orders, and if enough people ask for the tortillas, the store may start carrying them as a matter of course.

If even that fails, go online and do a search for "low-carbohydrate tortillas." You'll find plenty of e-tailers happy to ship them to you.

Low-carb tortillas are not exactly like either flour or corn tortillas; they have a flavor and texture of their own. We really enjoy them, and they sure are versatile! With a package of low-carb tortillas in the house and some cheese in the fridge, you've got a quick meal, any time.

I have tried making low-carb tortilla chips by cutting low-carb tortillas into wedges and frying them. The results were edible, but not great—tough, and a bit cardboards. Feel free to try it if you'd like. Me, I'd rather have nuts or fiber crackers or something.

Since I didn't like the low-carb tortilla chips, I haven't tried frying these low- carb tortillas to make taco shells or tostadas. I think the low-carb tortillas are best left in their original soft-and-pliable state. This chapter will teach you a few ways to use them.

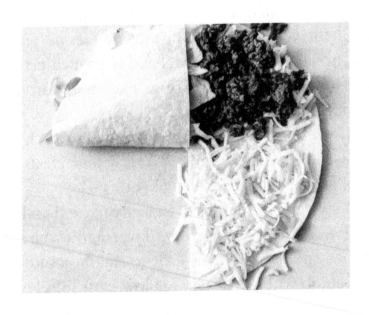

Gorgonzola and Pecan Quesadillas

This makes a casually elegant snack or starter for company, but it's too good not to make it just for yourself.

    1/4 cup (28 g) chopped pecans
    2 teaspoons butter, divided
    1/2 teaspoon Cajun seasoning
    3 ounces (85 g) crumbled gorgonzola cheese
    2 low carb tortillas, large

Over medium-low heat, sauté the pecans in the butter, stirring often, until they smell toasty. Stir in the Cajun seasoning and remove from the heat before they can scorch!

In a big skillet over medium heat, lay one tortilla flat, spread the crumbled gorgonzola evenly over it, and then layer in the pecans. Top with the second

tortilla. Let it cook 4 to 5 minutes and then flip carefully. Give it another 3 to 4 minutes. Cut into quarters to remove from the skillet.

Yield: 2 servings, each with 367 calories, 29 grams fat, 10 grams protein, 24 grams carbohydrate, 17 grams dietary fiber, and 7 grams usable carb.

Tortilla Pizza

This makes a great snack or light lunch. Keep in mind that the sauce is the highest carb part of this; don't go increasing the quantity.

> 1 low-carb tortilla
> 1 1/2 tablespoons (23 g) no-sugar-added pizza sauce 1/2 cup (60 g) shredded mozzarella cheese

Place the tortilla on the baking tray of the toaster oven. Spread the pizza sauce over it and then top with the cheese. Bake in the toaster oven at 450°F (230°C, or gas mark 8) until the cheese is bubbly and starting to brown (about 5 minutes). Cut into wedges and devour, watching out for pizza burns!

If you don't have a toaster oven, you have a couple of options: You can make the pizza in a conventional oven, but it will take a while to get up to 450°F (230°C, gas mark 8). You can cook it in a dry skillet, like an open-faced quesadilla —but you won't flip it, of course! This will melt the cheese, especially if you cover the pan with a tilted lid, but the cheese won't brown. If I were doing it this way, I'd cook it until the cheese was just melting and then put the whole skillet under the broiler for a minute to brown the cheese.

(Make sure your skillet has an ovenproof handle, if you decide to do this.) Or you could just put the pizza sauce and cheese on half of the tortilla and fold it over like a quesadilla.

Yield: 1 serving, with 16 grams of carbohydrates and 9 grams of fiber, for a total of 7 grams of usable carbs (you can drop it a little lower by using really low-carb pizza sauce) and 18 grams of protein.

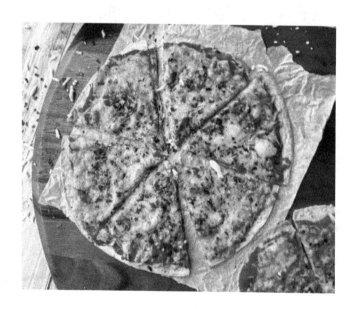

15-Minute Burgers

When we first discussed this project, my editor, Holly, and I discussed recipes that simply wouldn't work for the 15-minute framework. Holly brought up meat loaves. "Hah!" I said. "I'll just make them as burgers."

And that's what I've done. Here, for your quick-cooking, low-carbing pleasure, is an astonishing variety of interesting burger recipes, not a few of which originated as high-carb meat loaf recipes.

All of these recipes assume that you have an electric tabletop grill—you know, the George Foreman kind of thing. Since these grills cook from both sides, they cook very rapidly. If you don't have one, no worries—there's no reason you can't cook these burgers in a skillet or even broil them—it'll just take an extra 5 minutes or so, and you'll have to flip them.

By the way, you'll find a number of burger recipes here that use pork. If you don't eat pork, I don't see any reason why ground turkey wouldn't work in these recipes. It would taste different, but should still taste good. If you do this, chop all of your other ingredients in a food processor and then add the ground turkey and pulse just long enough to combine.

Apple Sausage Burgers

Feel free to make these with turkey sausage, if you prefer.

> 1/2 medium onion, peeled and cut in a few chunks
>
> 1/2 Granny Smith or other crisp, tart apple, cut into a few chunks (no need to peel it)
>
> 1 1/2 pounds (680 g) bulk pork sausage, hot or mild
>
> 1 teaspoon dried thyme
>
> 1 teaspoon dried sage 1 teaspoon pepper

Preheat your electric tabletop grill.

Put the onion and apple in a food processor with the S-blade in place and pulse until they're chopped to a medium consistency. Add the sausage, thyme, sage, and pepper and pulse until it's all well-blended.

Form into 4 burger and put them on the grill. Cook for 7 minutes or until the juices run clear.

Yield: 4 servings, each with 7 grams of carbohydrates and 1 gram of fiber, for a total of 6 grams of usable carbs and 20 grams of protein.

Apple Cheddar Pork Burgers

What can I say? I think apples and pork are a terrific combination.

> 1/2 Granny Smith or other crisp, tart apple, cut into a few chunks (no need to peel it)
> 1/4 medium onion, peeled and cut into a couple of chunks
> 1 pound (455 g) boneless pork loin, cut into 1 1/2
> 1 egg
> 1/2 teaspoon salt or Vege-Sal
> 2 teaspoons prepared horseradish
> 2 ounces (55 g) cheddar cheese, shredded

Preheat your electric tabletop grill.

Put the apple, onion, pork, oat bran, egg, salt or Voge-Sal, and horseradish in a food processor and pulse until the meat is ground and everything is well- blended. Add the cheese and pulse just long enough to blend it in—we're trying to keep some actual shreds of cheese here.

Form into 4 burgers and slap 'em on the grill. Cook for 7 minutes or until the juices run clear.

Yield: 4 servings, each with 5 grams of carbohydrates and 1 gram of fiber, for a total of 4 grams of usable carbs and 25 grams of protein.

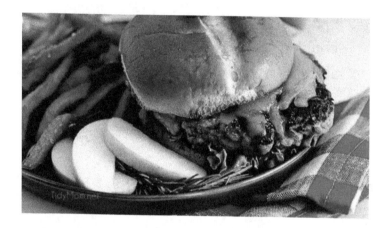

Ham and Pork Burgers

These are sort of plain and simple, but my husband loves them. This is a good recipe to help you use up leftover ham, should you have any on hand — but of course, you can also buy a chunk of precooked ham at the grocery store.

> 1/2 pound (225 g) cooked ham, cut into chunks
> 3/4 pound (340 g) boneless pork loin, cut into chunks
> 2 tablespoons (12 g) oat bran
> 2 tablespoons (28 ml) heavy cream
> 1 egg
> 1/2 teaspoon pepper

Preheat your electric tabletop grill.

Plunk the ham, pork loin, oat bran, cream, egg, and pepper in a food processor with the **S**-blade in place and pulse until the meat is finely ground. Form into 4 burgers and put them in the grill. Cook for 6 to 7 minutes and serve.

Yield: 4 servings, each with no more than 5 grams of carbohydrates (less, if you use really low-carb ham) and 1 gram of fiber, for a total of no more than 4 grams of usable carbs and 28 grams of protein.

Orange Lamb Burgers

Don't bother grinding your own lamb in your food processor; I tried this, and it came out a bit gristly. Buy ground lamb, instead. If you can't find ground lamb at your grocery store, ask the nice meat guy.

1/4 large sweet red onion
2 cloves garlic or 1 teaspoon minced garlic
1 pound (455 g) ground lamb
1 teaspoon ground cumin
1 1/2 tablespoons (23 ml) soy sauce
2 teaspoons grated orange zest
2 tablespoons (28 ml) orange juice
2 tablespoons (2 g) chopped cilantro
1/4 teaspoon salt
1/2 teaspoon pepper

Preheat your electric tabletop grill.

Either chop the red onion and the garlic to a medium-fine consistency in your food processor using the **S**-blade or cut 'em up with a knife. Then put them and the lamb, cumin, soy sauce, orange zest, orange juice, cilantro, salt, and pepper in a big bowl. Using clean hands, smoosh everything together until it's all very well blended. Form the mixture into 4 burgers and put them on the grill. Cook for 7 minutes and serve.

Yield: 4 servings, each with 3 grams of carbohydrates, a trace of fiber, and 20 grams of protein.

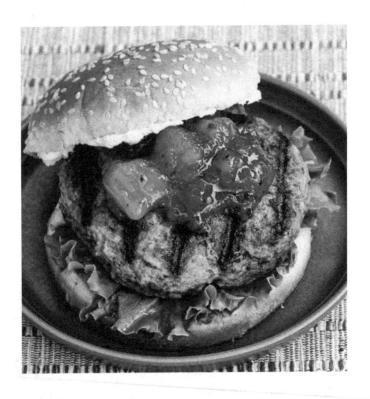

Mediterranean Lamb Burgers

This is about as upscale as a cheeseburger can get. My husband, who generally prefers beef to lamb, thought these were great.

1/4 medium onion

2 tablespoons (7 g) sun-dried tomatoes

1 pound (455 g) ground lamb

1 tablespoon (15 g) jarred pesto sauce

1 tablespoon (10 g) chopped garlic

1/4 teaspoon pepper

1/2 teaspoon salt or Vege-Sal

2 tablespoons (18 g) pine nuts

3 ounces (85 g) chèvre (goat) cheese

Preheat your electric tabletop grill; I set mine to 350°F (180°C).

Chop your onion and if your sun-dried tomatoes are in halves rather than prechopped, chop them up, too. Heck, even if they're prechopped, chop them a little more. Throw these things in a mixing bowl.

Add the ground lamb, pesto, garlic, pepper, and salt. Use clean hands to squish it all together until it's well-mixed. Form into three patties and throw them in the grill. Set a timer for 5 minutes.

While the burgers are cooking, toast your pine nuts until they're touched with gold.

When your burgers are done, plate them, crumble an ounce (28 g) of chèvre over each one, sprinkle with pine nuts, and then serve.

Yield: 3 servings, each with 578 calories, 47 grams fat, 33 grams protein, 4 grams carbohydrate, 1 gram dietary fiber, and 3 grams usable carb.

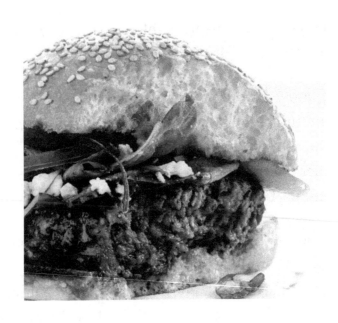

Thai Burgers

Boy are these good! If you can't find fish sauce, you can substitute soy sauce and this will still taste fine.

> 1 1/2 pounds (680 g) boneless pork loin, cut into chunks
> 1 1/2 teaspoons lemon juice
> 1 tablespoon (16 g) chili garlic paste
> 1 clove garlic or 1/2 teaspoon minced garlic
> 4 scallions, with the roots and the tops cut off (leave the crisp part of the green!)
> 1 can 4 ounces, or (15 g) mushrooms, drained
>
> 1 tablespoon (15 ml) fish sauce
> 2 tablespoons (2 g) fresh cilantro
> 3 tablespoons (45 ml) lime juice
> 1/2 cup (115 g) mayonnaise (100 ml) Preheat

your electric tabletop grill.

Put the pork loin, lemon juice, garlic paste, garlic, scallions, mushrooms, fish sauce, and cilantro in a food processor with the S-blade in place. Pulse until the meat is finely ground and everything is well-combined. Form the mixture into 6 burgers and put them on the grill. Cook for 6 to 7 minutes.

While the burgers are cooking, stir the lime juice (bottled works fine) into the mayonnaise. When the burgers are done, top each one with a dollop of the lime mayonnaise and serve.

Yield: 6 servings, each with 4 grams of carbohydrates and 1 gram of fiber, for a total of 3 grams of usable carbs and 24 grams of protein.

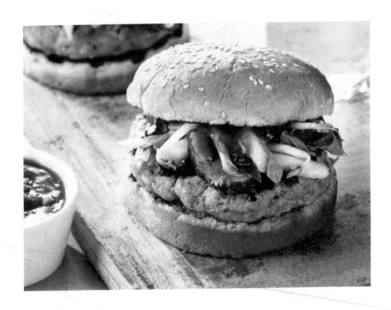

Banh Mi Burgers

I saw a recipe for a Vietnamese meatball sandwich and thought, "I could make that into burgers." So I did. For a full meal, make the *Hot and Sweet Mostly Asian Slaw* and serve the burgers and sauce on top of the slaw. But these are tasty even without the slaw!

> 5 scallions, divided
> 1/4 (15 g) cup fresh basil leaves
> 1 pound (455 g) ground pork
> 2 teaspoons chopped garlic
> 1 tablespoon (20 g) fish sauce
> 1 tablespoon (20 g) Sriracha chili sauce
> 1 tablespoon (1.5 g) Splenda, or its equivalent in sweetness 1 teaspoon salt
> 1 teaspoon pepper
> 1/3 cup (75 g) mayonnaise
> 1 tablespoon (20 g) Sriracha chili sauce

Preheat electric tabletop grill. If you can choose temperature settings on yours, use 350°F (180°C).

Cut the root and any limp greens off the scallions, whack them into a few pieces, and throw three of them into your food processor with the S-blade in place. (Reserve the other two.) Throw in the basil, too. Pulse until they're finely chopped together.

Now add ingredients from the pork through the pepper and run the processor until it's all well-blended.

Make the pork mixture into three patties and put them in the grill. Set a timer for 6 to 8 minutes.

Quickly wash out your food processor and reassemble with the S-blade in place. Put the remaining scallions in there and pulse to chop. Now add the mayo and chili sauce and run to blend.

When the burgers are done, serve with the sauce.

Yield: 3 servings, each with 597 calories, 53 grams fat, 27 grams protein, 5 grams carbohydrate, 1 gram dietary fiber, and 4 grams usable carb.

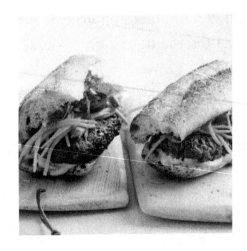

Luau Burgers

Again, all those ingredients make this look intimidating, but it's really just a matter of assembling everything in the food processor and chopping it together.

1 pound (455 g) boneless pork loin

1/4 medium onion, cut into chunks

1/2 green pepper, cut into chunks

1 1/2 teaspoons grated ginger-root

1/2 teaspoon minced garlic or 1 clove garlic, crushed 1 tablespoon (15 ml) soy sauce

1 egg

1/4 cup (60 g) crushed pork rinds, plain or barbeque flavor

1/2 teaspoon pepper

1/2 teaspoon salt

1/4 cup (60 g) canned crushed pineapple in unsweetened juice 1 tablespoon (15 g) tomato sauce

1/2 teaspoon blackstrap molasses

1/2 teaspoon Splenda

1/2 teaspoon spicy brown mustard

Preheat your electric tabletop grill.

Place the pork, onion, pepper, gingerroot, garlic, soy sauce, egg, pork rinds, pepper, and salt in a food processor with the S-blade in place. (You'll need a full-size food processor; this overwhelmed my little one!) Pulse until the meat is finely ground. Add the pineapple and pulse to mix.

Form into 5 burgers—the mixture will be quite soft—and slap them on the grill. Set a timer for 6 minutes.

While the burgers are cooking, mix together the tomato sauce, molasses, Splenda, and mustard. When the 6 minutes are up, open the grill, spread the tomato sauce mixture evenly over the burgers, and then close the grill and cook for 1 more minute. Serve.

Yield: 5 servings, each with 5 grams of carbohydrates and 1 gram of fiber, for a total of 4 grams of usable carbs and 22 grams of protein.These are low calorie, too! Just 178 calories perserving.

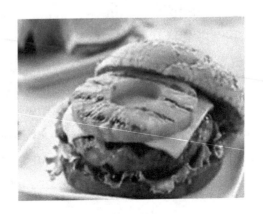

Chili Burgers

Here's all the long-simmered flavor of chili in a fast-and-easy burger.

    1 pound (455 g) ground beef
    1 cup (241 g) canned tomatoes with green chilies
    1/2 medium onion, finely minced
    2 cloves garlic, crushed
    1 tablespoon (8 g) chili powder
    2 tablespoons (30 g) crushed barbecue-flavor
       pork rinds
    1 tablespoon (16g) tomato paste
    1 tablespoon (18 g) salt or Vege-Sal
    4 ounces (115 g) cheddar cheese, sliced Sour
    cream (optional)

Preheat your electric tabletop grill.

Plunk the beef, tomatoes, onion, garlic, chili powder, pork rinds, tomato paste, and salt into a bowl and using clean hands, smoosh it all together until everything is thoroughly combined. Form this mixture into 4 patties, put them

on the grill, and cook for 5 minutes.

When the 5 minutes are up, open your grill but do not remove the burgers. Top each with a slice of cheddar cheese and use whatever heatproof kitchen object you have on hand to prop the lid of the grill open slightly for a minute or so. Let the cheese melt and serve with a dollop of sour cream, if you like.

Yield: 4 servings, each with 6 grams of carbohydrates and 1 gram of fiber, for a total of 5 grams of usable carbs and 28 grams of protein. Add 1 gram of carbs and 1 gram of protein if you use the sourcream.

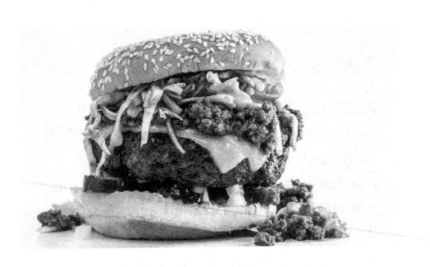

Crunchy Peking Burgers

1/2 cup (62 g) canned water chestnuts, drained

2 scallions

1 pound (455 g) ground beef

1/4 cup (60 ml) soy sauce

2 tablespoons (28 ml) dry sherry

1 teaspoon Splenda

1 teaspoon minced garlic or 2 cloves garlic, crushed 1/2 teaspoon grated gingerroot

Sauce

1 1/2 tablespoons (30 g) low-sugar apricot preserves 1 teaspoon soy sauce 1/4 teaspoon grated gingerroot

Preheat your electric tabletop grill.

Chop the water chestnuts a bit and slice the scallions. Put them in a mixing bowl with all the other burger ingredients and using clean hands, mix them well. Form into 4 burgers and put them on the grill. Cook for 5 minutes.

While the burgers are cooking, mix together the preserves, soy sauce, and gingerroot in a small dish. When the burgers are done, top each with a teaspoon of sauce and serve.

Yield: 4 servings, each with 7 grams of carbohydrates and 1 gram of fiber, for a total of 6 grams of usable carbs and 20 grams of protein.

15-Minute Poultry

You'll find that most of these recipes depend upon the ubiquitous boneless, skinless chicken breast. There's a reason for this: It's nearly impossible to cook chicken on the bone in 15 minutes or less! And even with boneless, skinless chicken breasts, it's helpful, in a fair number of recipes, to pound them a little to make them thinner and an even thickness all over. This is very easy to do and takes no more than 15 to 30 seconds per breast—time well spent if it cuts 5 minutes off the cooking time. Once you've beaten a chicken breast flat a few times, you'll wonder why you've never done it before.

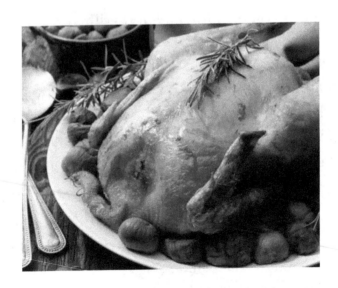

Singing Chicken

This is another Vietnamese dish, and it is definitely for those who enjoy breathing fire. I'm a big fan of hot food, and this dish had me sweating by halfway through the meal. Delicious! It's droccoli goes nicely with this.

> 1 to 3 tablespoons (28 to 45 ml) vegetable oil, preferably peanut
>
> 1 tablespoon (8 g) grated gingerroot
>
> 1 teaspoon minced garlic or 2 cloves garlic, crushed
>
> 1 1/2 pounds (680 g) boneless, skinless chicken breast, cut crosswise into thin slices*
>
> 2 tablespoons (3 g) Splenda
>
> 1/4 cup (60 ml) soy sauce
>
> 1 teaspoon fish sauce (nuoc mam)
>
> 3/4 cup (175 ml) dry white wine
>
> 1 fresh jalapeño, or 2 or 3 little red chilies, finely minced
>
> 1 teaspoon pepper
>
> Guar or xanthan

* This is easiest if the meat is half-frozen.

Have the chicken sliced, the ingredients measured, the pepper minced, and everything standing by and ready to go before starting to cook—once you start stir-frying, this goes very quickly.

Put a wok or heavy skillet over high heat. Add the oil, let it heat for a minute or so, and then add the ginger and garlic. Stir for 1 minute to flavor the oil. Add the chicken, and stir-fry for 1 to 2 minutes. Add the Splenda, soy sauce, fish sauce, white wine, jalapeño, and pepper, stirring often, for 7 to 8 minutes

or until the chicken is cooked through. Thicken pan juices very slightly with guar or xanthan and serve.

Yield: 3 or 4 servings. Assuming 4 servings, each will have 4 grams of carbohydrates, a trace of fiber, and 39 grams of protein.

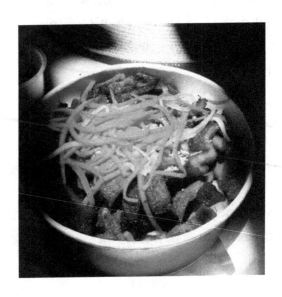

Crispy Skillet BBQ Chicken

Add some slaw made from bagged coleslaw mix, and supper is served.

> 1 1/2 pounds (680 g) boneless, skinless chicken breast Sprinkle-on barbecue dry rub or "soul" seasoning
> 1/2 cup (120 g) crushed barbecue-flavor pork rinds
> 2 tablespoons (28 ml) oil

One at a time, pound the chicken breasts until they're about 1/2 inch (1.3 cm) thick all over. If necessary, cut the breasts into 4 servings. Sprinkle both sides of each piece liberally with the seasoning. Then sprinkle each side of each serving with 1 tablespoon (15 g) of the pork rind crumbs and press them onto the surface with a clean palm.

Heat the oil in a large, heavy-bottomed skillet over medium-high heat. Add the chicken breasts and sauté for 5 to 6 minutes per side or until crispy and cooked through. Serve. This is great with any sort of salad or coleslaw as a side.

Yield: 4 servings. This has no carbs to speak of (maybe a tiny trace from the seasoning), no fiber, and 44 grams of protein per serving.

Aegean Chicken

The minute I told my sister about this, she started hounding me for the recipe.

1 1/2 pounds (680 g) boneless, skinless chicken breast

1/4 cup (60 ml) olive oil

4 ounces (115 g) kasseri cheese, sliced

8 tablespoons (64 g) tapenade

1/4 cup (60 ml) dry white wine

2 cloves garlic

One at a time, pound the chicken breasts till they're 1/4 inch (6 mm) thick all over. Cut the breasts into 6 servings, if necessary. Sauté them in the olive oil over medium-high heat. When they're turning golden on the bottom, turn them and lay the slices of kasseri over them. Let them cook another 2 to 3 minutes or until the cheese is starting to melt. Spread the tapenade over the breasts and add the wine to the skillet. Let the whole thing cook for another minute or two, just to warm the tapenade and make sure the chicken is cooked through. Remove the chicken to serving plates, add the garlic to the wine left in the skillet, stir the whole thing and let it boil for a minute or so, and pour it over the chicken before serving.

Yield: 6 servings, each with just 2 grams of carbohydrates, a trace of fiber, and 40 grams of protein.

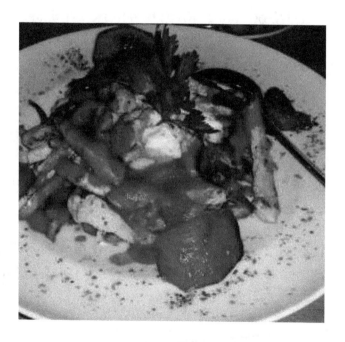

Cashew Crusted Chicken

Since cashews are a relatively high-carb nut, this is just a light coating—but very flavorful. You can find raw cashews at most health food stores.

  2/3 cup (93 g) raw cashew pieces
  1/4 teaspoon salt
  1/2 teaspoon pepper
  1/4 teaspoon paprika
  1 1/2 pounds (680 g) boneless, skinless chicken breast 1 egg
  2 to 3 tablespoons (28 to 42 g) butter

First, put the cashew pieces in a food processor with the S-blade in place and grind them to a fine texture. Dump them out onto a plate and add the salt, pepper, and paprika, mixing the whole thing well. Set aside.

Pound the chicken breasts until they're 1/2 inch (1.3 cm) thick all over. Cut into 4 servings if necessary.

Break the egg into another plate with a rim around it. (A pie plate would work well.) Now, dip each chicken breast piece into the egg, then into the cashew mixture, coating both sides.

Melt the butter in a heavy skillet over medium to medium-high heat and add the chicken. Sauté until it's golden on both sides and cooked through, about 5

minutes per side.

Yield: 4 servings, each with 6 grams of carbohydrates and 1 gram of fiber, for a total of 5 grams of usable carbs and 33 grams of protein.

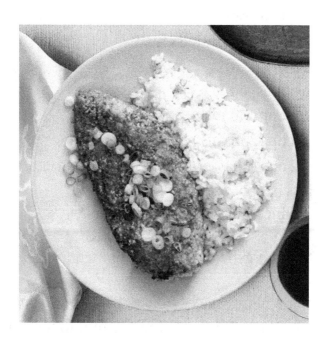

Almond Chicken with Gorgonzola Cream Sauce

This dish is simply fantastic—lush and creamy and decadent. It's just fantastic. Do pound the chicken out thin enough, though, or it'll take an extra few minutes.

1 pound (455 g) boneless, skinless chicken breast
1 tablespoon (14 g) butter
1 tablespoon (15 ml) olive oil
1 cup (112 g) almond meal
2 tablespoons (16 g) coconut flour
1/2 teaspoon salt or Vege-Sal
1/4 teaspoon pepper
1 teaspoon ground sage
1 egg
1 tablespoon (15 ml) water
1/4 cup (60 ml) dry white wine
 1 cup (235 ml) heavy cream
1/2 cup (60 g) crumbled gorgonzola cheese salt and pepper
2 tablespoons (3 g) minced parsley

Set your big, heavy skillet over medium heat.

Using a blunt, heavy object, beat your chicken breast out to 1/4 to 1/3 inch (6 mm to 8 mm) thick. Cut into four portions.

On a plate with a rim, combine the almond meal, coconut flour, salt, pepper, and sage. On another plate, beat up the egg with the water.

Add the butter and olive oil to the skillet and slosh them around.

Dip each piece of chicken in the egg on both sides, then the almond meal mixture. Lay them in the skillet and cover with a tilted lid.

While the chicken is cooking, measure out the wine, cream, and gorgonzola.

Okay, chicken's golden on one side. Flip it and cook the other, again, with the tilted lid over it.

When the chicken's done, plate it and keep it warm.

Add the wine to the skillet and crank the heat up to high. Boil it down for a minute and then add the cream and the gorgonzola. Let the sauce boil hard, stirring constantly until it's reduced and thickened a bit. You can add a little guar, xanthan, or glucomannan if you like. Salt and pepper the sauce, spoon it over the chicken, top with parsley, and serve.

Yield: 4 servings, each with 645 calories, 43 grams fat, 46 grams protein, 18 grams carbohydrate, 4 grams dietary fiber, and 14 grams usable carb.

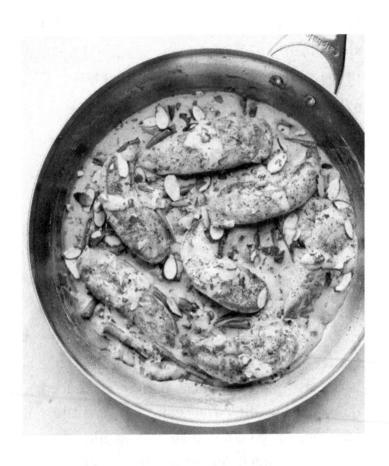

Chicken Breast Italiano

This dish is ridiculously easy, especially considering how good it tastes! It's great with one of the cauliflower "risottos" as a side dish.

> 1 1/2 pounds (680 g) boneless, skinless chicken breast
> 2 tablespoons (28 ml) olive oil
> 1/3 cup (80 ml) bottled Italian salad dressing

In a heavy-bottomed skillet, sauté the chicken breasts in the olive oil over medium heat. Cover them while they're cooking and turn them after 6 to 7 minutes. When both sides are golden and the chicken is cooked most of the way through, add the Italian dressing, turn the breasts to coat both sides, and let the whole thing cook for another 2 to 3 minutes before serving.

Yield: 4 servings, each with 2 grams of carbohydrates, no fiber, and 38 grams of protein.

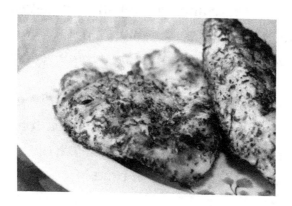

Chicken Tenders

This is good for when you're having fast-food cravings or the kids are nagging for "normal" food. You really can make these in 15 minutes—because the pieces are small, they cook very quickly.

> 1 pound (455 g) boneless, skinless chicken breast 1 egg
> 1 tablespoon (15 ml) water
> 3/4 cup (94 g) low-carb bake mix
> 1/2 teaspoon salt
> 1/4 teaspoon pepper
> 1/3 cup (80 ml) oil

Cut the chicken breasts into pieces about 1 inch (2.5 cm) wide and 2 inches (5 cm) long. Beat the egg with the water in a bowl. On a plate, combine the bake mix with the salt and pepper. Heat the oil in a heavy skillet over medium-high heat.

Dip each chicken piece in the egg wash, then roll it in the seasoned bake mix, and drop it in the hot oil. Fry these until golden all over and serve with one of the dipping sauces in the *Condiments, Sauces, Dressings, and Seasonings* chapter.

Yield: 4 servings, each with 5 grams of carbohydrates and 2 grams of fiber, for a total of 3 grams of usable carbs (exclusive of the dipping sauces) and 40 grams of protein.

Seriously Spicy Citrus Chicken

You could cut back on the red pepper flakes if you'd like to make Moderately Spicy Citrus Chicken.

1 1/2 pounds (680 g) boneless, skinless chicken breast
1/4 cup (60 ml) olive oil
1/2 cup (120 ml) lime juice
1/4 cup (60 ml) lemon juice
1 tablespoon (4 g) plus
1 teaspoon (1 g) red pepper flakes
1 tablespoon (6 g) plus
1 teaspoon (2 g) minced garlic
1 tablespoon (8 g) plus
1 teaspoon (3 g) grated ginger root
1/4 cup (6 g) Splenda
4 scallions, finely sliced
2 tablespoons (2 g) chopped cilantro

Cut the chicken into 4 servings, if necessary. Sauté the chicken in the olive oil over medium-high heat, with a tilted lid. While it's sautéing, mix together the lime juice, lemon juice, red pepper flakes, garlic, gingerroot, and Splenda. After the chicken has turned golden on both sides (about 4 to 5 minutes per side), pour the lime juice mixture into the skillet and turn the breasts over to coat both sides. Sauté for another 2 to 3 minutes on each side and then move the chicken to serving plates, scraping the liquid from the pan over the chicken. Scatter sliced scallions and chopped cilantro over each portion and serve.

Yield: 4 servings, each with 8 grams of carbohydrates and 1 gram of fiber, for a total of 7 grams of usable carbs and 32 grams of protein.

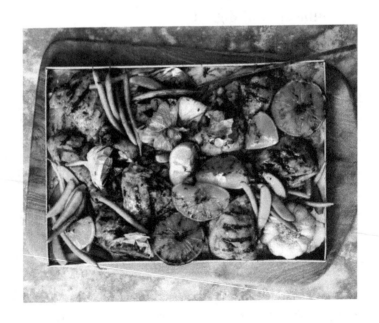

Lemon-Herb Chicken Breast

This dish is simple and classic and summery.

> 1 teaspoon chopped garlic
> 1/2 cup (120 ml) olive oil
> 1 pound (455 g) boneless, skinless chicken
> breast salt and pepper
> 1/4 cup (10 g) minced fresh basil
> 2 tablespoons (5 g) minced fresh parsley
> 2 lemons
> 2 tablespoons (28 ml) water

Put the garlic in a measuring cup and pour the olive oil over it. Let it sit. Give a skillet a squirt of nonstick cooking spray and put it over a high burner.

Now grab your chicken and a blunt, heavy object and pound your breast out to an even 1/2 inch (1.3 cm) thickness. Cut into three portions and salt and pepper it on both sides.

Pour half or so of the garlicky olive oil into your now-hot skillet, slosh it around, and throw in your chicken. Cover it with a tilted lid and let it cook for 3 to 4 minutes.

Mince your basil and parsley. Also roll your lemon under your palm, pressing down firmly. This will help it render more juice.

Your chicken should be golden on the bottom now; flip it! Re-cover with the tilted lid and give it another 3 to 4 minutes. In the meantime, slice your lemon in half and flick out the seeds with the tip of a knife.

When your chicken is golden on both sides, squeeze one of the lemons over it. Flip it to coat both sides, turn the burner down to medium low, and re- cover with that tilted lid. Let it cook until it's done through.

Plate your chicken and then add the water and the juice of the other lemon to the skillet. Stir it all around with a fork, scraping up the tasty brown bits, and then pour this over the chicken. Top with the herbs and a last drizzle of garlic olive oil and then serve.

Yield: 3 servings, each with 508 calories, 40 grams fat, 34 grams protein, 5 grams carbohydrate, 1 gram dietary fiber, and 4 grams usable carb.

Apricot-Bourbon Chicken

This is amazing—as good as anything I've ever had in a fancy restaurant—yet it's fast enough to make on a weeknight after work! I like the *Saffron "Rice"* as a side with this.

> 2 pounds (900 g) boneless, skinless chicken breasts 3 tablespoons (42 g) butter
> 1/2 cup (55 g) chopped pecans
> 1/4 cup (80 g) low-sugar apricot preserves
> 1/4 cup (60 ml) bourbon
> 2 tablespoons (31 g) plain tomato sauce
> 2 teaspoons spicy brown or Dijon mustard
> 1/2 teaspoon minced garlic or 1 clove garlic, crushed 1/4 cup (40 g) minced onion
> 3 scallions, thinly sliced

First, pound the chicken breasts until they're 1/2 inch (1.3 cm) thick all over and cut into 6 portions. Brown them in 2 tablespoons (28 g) of butter in a large, heavy skillet over high heat.

While the breasts are browning, melt the last tablespoon (14 g) of butter in a small, heavy skillet and stir in the pecans. Stir them over medium-high heat for a few minutes until they begin to turn golden. Turn off the heat (and if yours is an electric stove, remove from the burner to prevent scorching) and reserve.

Stir together the preserves, bourbon, tomato sauce, mustard, garlic, and onion.

When the chicken is light golden on both sides, pour this mixture into the skillet. Turn the chicken over once or twice to coat both sides with the sauce. Cover with a tilted lid and let it simmer for about 5 minutes or until cooked through.

Serve with the sauce spooned over each portion and top each with the toasted pecans and sliced scallions.

Yield: 6 servings, each with 7 grams of carbohydrates and 1 gram of fiber, for a total of 6 grams of usable carbs and 35 grams of protein.

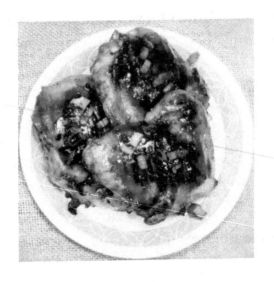

Chicken Breasts L'Orange

Chicken combines so well with all sorts of fruit flavors, and this dish is sure to be a hit with the whole family.

> 1 1/2 pounds (680 g) boneless, skinless chicken breast 1/4 cup (60 ml) oil
> 1/3 cup (80 ml) orange juice
> 2 tablespoons
> (3 g) Splenda
> 2 teaspoons cider vinegar
> 1/4 teaspoon blackstrap molasses
> 1 teaspoon spicy brown or Dijon mustard
> 1 teaspoon minced garlic or 2 cloves garlic, crushed Salt and pepper

Cut the chicken breasts into 4 portions and brown them in the oil in a large, heavy skillet over high heat. While that's happening, mix together the orange juice, Splenda, vinegar, molasses, mustard, and garlic. When the chicken is light golden on both sides, add the orange juice mixture to the skillet. Simmer the chicken for another 7 to 8 minutes, turning once. Salt and pepper to taste and serve.

Yield: 4 servings, each with 4 grams of carbohydrates, a trace of fiber, and 38 grams of protein.

Chicken with Asparagus and Gruyere

1 1/2 pounds (680 g) boneless, skinless
chicken breast 1 tablespoon (14 g) butter
1 pound (455 g) asparagus
1 tablespoon (15 ml) dry white wine
1 tablespoon (15 ml) lemon juice Salt and
pepper
4 ounces (115 g) gruyere cheese, thinly sliced

First, pound the chicken breasts until they're 1/4 inch (6 mm) thick all over. Cut into 4 portions.

Melt the butter in a large, heavy skillet over medium-high heat and start browning the chicken.

While that's happening, snap the ends off the asparagus where they break naturally. Put the asparagus in a microwaveable casserole or lay it in a glass pie plate. Add a couple of tablespoons (28 ml) of water and cover. (Use plastic wrap or a plate to cover if you're using a pie plate.) Microwave on High for 3 to 4 minutes.

When the chicken is golden on both sides, add the wine and the lemon juice to the skillet and turn the chicken breasts to coat both sides. Salt and pepper lightly. Turn the burner to medium-low heat and let the chicken continue to cook until the asparagus is done microwaving.

Remove the asparagus from the microwave and drain. Lay the asparagus spears over the chicken, dividing equally between the portions. Cover each with gruyere and cover the skillet with a tilted lid. Continue cooking a few minutes, just until the cheese is melted. Serve.

Yield: 4 servings, each with 3 grams of carbohydrates and 1 gram of fiber, for a total of 2 grams of usable carbs and 38 grams of protein.

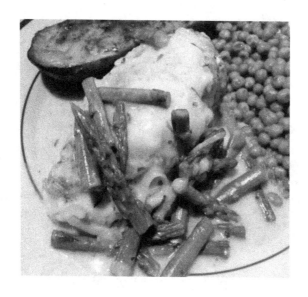

15-Minute Fish and Seafood

If you're trying to eat low-carb and to be as healthy as possible on a tight schedule, you just can't do any better than fish. Of course we know fish is wonderful for us, but it's also to our advantage that it's hard to find a fish recipe that calls for more than 15 minutes'cooking time!

Indeed, the only thing I can think of to say against fish is that it is often expensive. Around here, the fish we eat most often are catfish, tilapia, and whiting, for the simple reason that they're the fish that are cheapest, at least here in the Midwest.

However, fish are frequently interchangeable in recipes, so if you prefer sole, orange roughy, cod, flounder, or what-have-you, don't hesitate to try them. There's no reason why they shouldn't work out fine, with a little adjustment of time for thicker or thinner fillets.

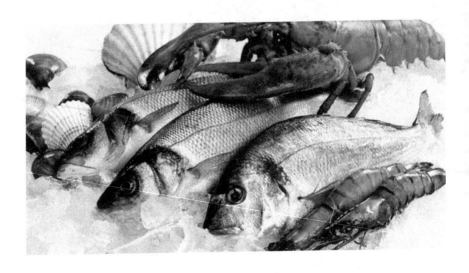

Saigon Shrimp

There are vietnamese style—hot and a little sweet.

Scant 1/2 teaspoon salt Scant
1/2 teaspoon pepper
1 1/2 teaspoons Splenda
3 scallions
4 tablespoons (60 ml) peanut or canola oil
1 pound (455 g) large shrimp, shelled and deveined
1 1/2 teaspoons chili garlic paste
2 teaspoons minced garlic

Mix together the salt, pepper, and Splenda in a small dish or cup. Slice the scallions thinly and set them aside. Gather all the ingredients except the scallions together—the actual cooking of this dish is lightning fast!

In a wok or heavy skillet over highest heat, heat the oil. Add the shrimp and stir-fry for 2 to 3 minutes or until they're about two-thirds pink. Add the chili garlic paste and garlic and keep stir-frying. When the shrimp are pink all over and all the way through, sprinkle the salt, pepper, and Splenda mixture over them and stir for just another 10 seconds or so. Turn off the heat and divide the shrimp between 3 serving plates. Top each serving with a scattering of sliced scallion and serve.

Yield: 3 servings, each with 2 grams of carbohydrates and 1 gram of fiber, for a total of 1 gram of usable carbs and 25 grams of protein.

This dish comes in at a low 288 calories a serving.

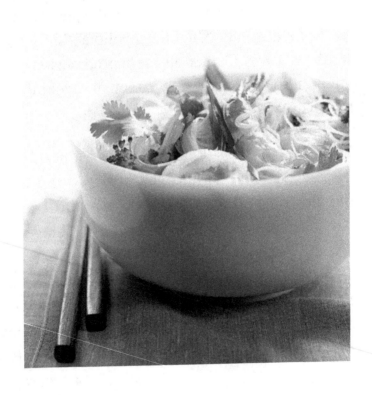

Basil-Lime Shrimp

1/2 cup (120 ml) lime juice

1/2 cup (120 ml) olive oil

1/4 cup (10 g) fresh basil — Just compact sprigs into your measuring cup.

4 teaspoons (16 g) brown mustard

1/4 teaspoon Splenda

4 scallions — thinly sliced, including the crisp part of the green

1/2 pound (225 g) shrimp

Put everything from the lime juice through the Splenda in your blender and

run it just for a second or two. Pour the mixture into a big nonreactive pan and place over medium heat. Bring to a simmer, turn the heat down to keep it just simmering, and let it cook until it's reduced by about half. While that's happening, slice your scallions.

When the lime juice mixture is reduced, lay the shrimp in it, in one layer if possible. (If not, you'll have to stir them around some.) Let them poach for about two minutes and then flip and give them another couple of minutes, just until they're firm and pink. Serve drizzled with the sauce, with the sliced scallion sprinkled over the top.

Yield: 4 servings, each with 438 calories, 30 grams fat, 35 grams protein, 6 grams carbohydrate, 1 gram dietary fiber, and 5 grams usable carb.

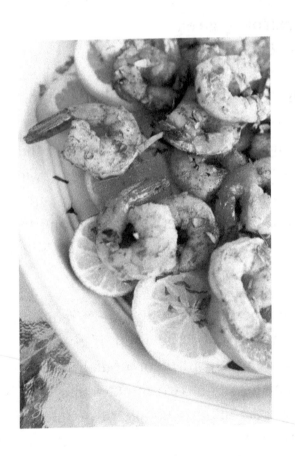

Shrimp in Brandy Cream

Wow—this is sheer elegance. And it's done in a flash!

> 1 pound (455 g) shrimp, shelled and deveined
> 4 tablespoons (55 g) butter
> 1/3 cup (80 ml) brandy
> 3/4 cup (175 ml) heavy cream Guar or xanthan (optional)

Sauté the shrimp in the butter over medium-high heat until cooked through— 4 to 5 minutes. Add the brandy, turn up the heat, and let it boil hard for a minute or so to reduce. Stir in the cream and heat through. Thicken the sauce a bit with guar or xanthan if you like and then serve.

Yield: 3 or 4 servings. Assuming 3 servings, each will have 2 grams of carbohydrates, no

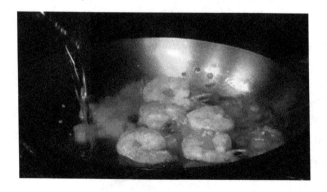

fiber, and 26 grams of protein.

Shrimp in Curried Coconut Milk

Coconut is emerging as a true super-food, and it certainly gives this dish a rich, exotic flavor. This is stew-like; serve it in bowls.

1/2 onion
1/2 green pepper
2 tablespoons (28 ml) coconut oil
2 teaspoons cumin
2 teaspoons curry powder
1 1/2 teaspoons ground coriander
1 1/2 teaspoons chopped garlic
1 cup (235 ml) unsweetened coconut milk
1/2 teaspoon salt or Vege-Sal
1/4 teaspoon chili garlic paste
3 cups (384) frozen cooked salad shrimp, thawed

Throw your onion and green pepper in the food processor and pulse until they're chopped fine. In a heavy-bottomed skillet, start them sautéing in the coconut oil over medium heat.

When the onion and pepper are starting to soften, throw in the spices. Sauté another few minutes, add the garlic, and give it just another minute.

Add the coconut milk and stir the whole thing up. Stir in the salt and chili garlic paste, too.

Now add the thawed, drained shrimp, stir it in, and turn the burner up a little. Simmer for a minute or two, thickening with a little guar, xanthan, or glucomannan if you think it needs it. Then serve—with spoons, to get all of the sauce!

Yield: 3 servings, each with 235 calories, 11 grams fat, 28 grams protein, 6 grams carbohydrate, 1 gram dietary fiber, and 5 grams usable carb.

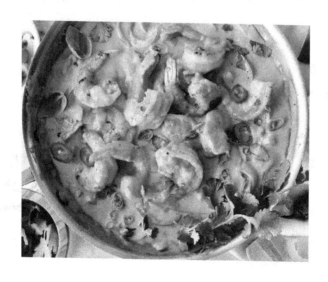

Salmon in Ginger Cream

This has all the goodness of salmon in an elegant sauce.

2 tablespoons (28 g) butter

2 pieces salmon fillet, 6 ounces (170 g) each, skin still attached 1 teaspoon minced garlic or 2 cloves garlic, crushed

2 scallions, finely minced

2 tablespoons (2 g) chopped cilantro

4 tablespoons (60 ml) dry white wine

2 tablespoons (16 g) grated ginger-root

4 tablespoons (60 g) sour cream Salt and pepper

Melt the butter in a heavy skillet over medium-low heat and start sautéing the salmon in it—you want to sauté it for about 4 minutes per side.

While the fish is sautéing, crush the garlic, mince the scallions, and chop the cilantro.

When both sides of the salmon have sautéed for 4 minutes, add the wine to the skillet, cover, and let the fish cook an additional 2 minutes or so until done through. Remove the fish to serving plates.

Add the garlic, scallions, cilantro, and ginger to the wine and butter in the skillet, turn the burner up to medium-high, and let them cook for a minute or two. Add the sour cream, stir to blend, and salt and pepper to taste. Spoon the sauce over the fish and serve.

Yield: 2 servings, each with 5 grams of carbohydrates and 1 gram of fiber, for a total of 4 grams of usable carbs and 36 grams of protein This dish also has lots of EPA—the good fat that makes salmon so heart-healthy!

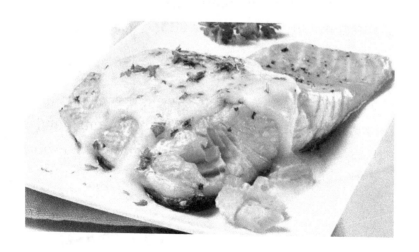

Buttered Salmon with Creole Seasonings

12 ounces (340 g) salmon fillet, in two or three
pieces
1 teaspoon purchased Creole seasoning
1/4 teaspoon dried thyme
4 tablespoons (55 g) butter
1 teaspoon minced garlic or 2 cloves garlic,
   minced

Sprinkle the skinless side of the salmon evenly with the Creole seasoning and thyme. Melt the butter in a heavy skillet over medium-low heat and add the salmon, skin side down. Cook 4 to 5 minutes per side, turning carefully. Remove to serving plates, skin side down, and stir the garlic into the butter remaining in the pan. Cook for just a minute, then scrape all the garlic butter over the salmon, and serve.

Yield: 2 or 3 servings. Assuming 2 servings, each will have 2 grams of carbohydrates and a trace of fiber, for a total of 2 grams of usable carbs and 35 grams of protein.

Glazed, Grilled Salmon

Of all the ways I've cooked salmon, this drew the most praise.

> 2 tablespoons (3 g) Splenda
> 1 1/2 teaspoons dry mustard
> 1 tablespoon (15 ml) soy sauce
> 1 1/2 teaspoons rice vinegar
> 1/4 teaspoon blackstrap molasses, or the darkest molasses you can find
> 12 ounces (340 g) salmon fillet, cut into 2 or 3 serving-size pieces

Mix together the Splenda, mustard, soy sauce, vinegar, and molasses in a small dish.

Spoon out 1 tablespoon (15 g) of this mixture and set it aside in a separate dish.

Place the salmon fillets on a plate and pour the larger quantity of the soy sauce mixture over it, turning each fillet so that both sides come in contact with the seasonings. Let the fish sit for a few minutes—just 2 or 3—with the skinless side down in the seasonings.

Now, you get to choose how you want to cook the salmon. I do mine on a stove top grill, but you can broil it, do it in a heavy skillet sprayed with nonstick cooking spray, cook it on your electric tabletop grill, or even do it on your outdoor grill. However you cook it, it will need about 5 minutes per side (or just 5 minutes total, in an electric grill). If you choose a method that requires you to turn the salmon, turn carefully! Baste once, when turning, with the soy sauce mixture you reserved. (Don't do it after that—you want the

heat to kill any raw fish germs!) When the salmon is cooked through, remove it to serving plates and drizzle the reserved seasoning mixture over each piece before serving.

Yield: This makes 2 generous servings or 3 smaller ones. Assuming 2 servings, each will have 3 grams of carbohydrates, a trace of fiber, and 35 grams of protein.

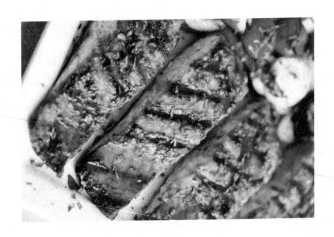

Peach Salmon

This makes a fruity-good summer supper.

> 24 ounces (680 g) salmon fillet in four servings
> 3 tablespoons (42 g) butter
> 2 fresh peaches
> 1/4 onion
> 1 teaspoon chopped garlic
> 1 1/2 teaspoons curry powder
> 2 tablespoons (28 ml) lemon juice
> 1/4 cup (6 g) Splenda or its equivalent in
> sweetness salt and pepper

Start the salmon sautéing in the butter over medium heat and cover it with a tilted lid.

Peel your peaches, halve, and remove the pits. Throw the peaches, onion, garlic, and curry powder in your food processor and pulse until the peach is chopped medium-fine. Go flip your salmon.

Mix together the lemon juice and Splenda. When your salmon is done through, plate it. Pour the lemon juice mixture in the skillet and stir it around, scraping up the yummy brown bits. Add the peach mixture and cook for just a minute or two, stirring. Salt and pepper to taste and then spoon over the salmon and serve.

Yield: 4 servings, each with 309 calories, 15 grams fat, 35 grams protein, 9 grams carbohydrate, 1 gram dietary fiber, and 8 grams usable carb.

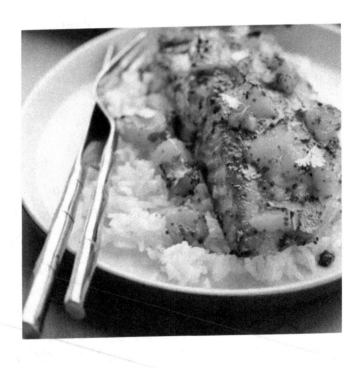

Salmon in Citrus Vinaigrette

My husband said this was perhaps the best salmon dish he'd ever had.

   1 tablespoon (15 ml) coconut oil
   24 ounces (680 g) salmon fillet in 4 servings
   1/2 cup (120 ml) vinaigrette (I used Paul
      Newman's light red wine vinegar and olive
      oil.) 1/2 cup (120 ml) lemon juice
   2 1/2 tablespoons (4 g) Splenda, or the
   equivalent in liquid Splenda
   1/4 teaspoon orange extract
   1 teaspoon brown mustard
   1 teaspoon chili powder
   2 tablespoons (28 ml) lime juice

Spray a big skillet with nonstick cooking spray and put it over medium heat. Throw in the coconut oil and when it's melted, slosh it around and then add the salmon.

While the salmon is getting a little touch of gold, throw everything else in the blender and run the thing.

Okay, go back and flip your salmon. Let it get a little gold on the other side, too.

Now add the vinaigrette mixture and turn the burner up to medium-high. Let the whole thing cook another five minutes or until the salmon is done through.

Plate the salmon and turn up the burner. Boil the vinaigrette hard until it's reduced and starting to get a little syrupy. Pour over the salmon and serve.

Yield: 4 servings, each with 384 calories, 25 grams fat, 34 grams protein, 5 grams carbohydrate, trace dietary fiber, and 5 grams usable carb.

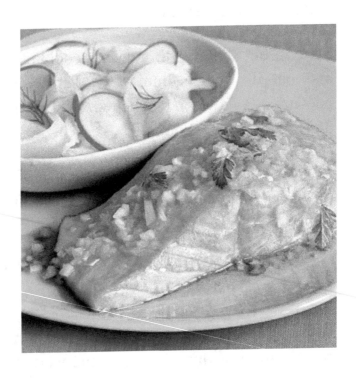

Skillet Barbecued Salmon

Don't panic at this list of ingredients; this really is quick and easy.

> 1/4 cup (115 g) bacon grease
>
> 24 ounces (680 g) salmon fillets, 1-inch (2.5 cm) thick and cut into four servings
>
> 2 tablespoons (28 ml) pineapple juice, or sugar-free pineapple syrup
>
> 1/4 cup (60 ml) soy sauce
>
> 1 1/3 tablespoons (20 ml) rice vinegar
>
> 1 1/3 tablespoons (20 ml) lemon juice
>
> 2 teaspoons olive oil
>
> 1/2 cup (12 g) Splenda
>
> 1/8 cup erythritol
>
> 1/3 teaspoon molasses
>
> 1/2 teaspoon pepper
>
> 1/3 teaspoon cayenne
>
> 1/3 teaspoon paprika
>
> 1/8 teaspoon garlic

Put your big, heavy skillet over medium-high heat and throw in the bacon grease. When it's hot, add the fillets. Let them sizzle there while you mix together everything else.

Flip your fillets after 4 to 5 minutes and let them get golden on the other side, too.

Now pour in the sauce and flip the fillets again to coat. Let them simmer in the sauce until they're done through. Then plate the fillets and turn up the burner. Boil the sauce until it's syrupy, pour over the fillets, and serve.

Yield: 4 servings, each with 366 calories, 21 grams fat, 35 grams protein, 7 grams carbohydrate, trace dietary fiber, and 7 grams usable carb.

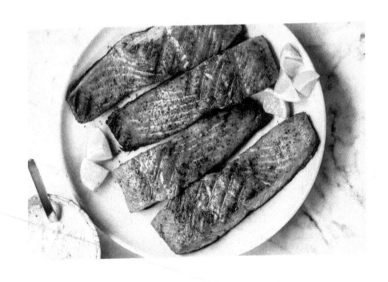

Whiting with Mexican Flavors

4 whiting fillets

2 tablespoons (28 ml) lime juice

3/4 teaspoon chili powder

2 tablespoons (28 ml) oil

1 medium onion

2 tablespoons (28 ml) orange juice

1/2 teaspoon Splenda

1/4 teaspoon ground cumin

1/4 teaspoon dried oregano

1 tablespoon (15 ml) white wine vinegar

1/2 teaspoon hot sauce

Salt and pepper

Lay the whiting fillets on a plate and sprinkle with 1 tablespoon (15 ml) of lime juice, turning to coat. Sprinkle the skinless sides of the fillets with chili powder.

Heat the oil in a heavy skillet over medium heat. Add the whiting fillets. Sauté for about 4 minutes per side, turning carefully, or until cooked through. Remove to a serving plate and keep warm.

Add the onions to the skillet and turn the heat up to medium-high. Sauté the onions for a couple of minutes until they begin to go limp. Stir in the orange juice, Splenda, cumin, oregano, vinegar, and hot sauce. Cook them all together for a minute or two. Salt and pepper to taste. Spoon the onions over the fish and serve.

Yield: 4 servings, each with 5 grams of carbohydrates and 1 gram of fiber, for a total of 4 grams of usable carbs and 17 grams of protein.

Each serving has only 162 calories!

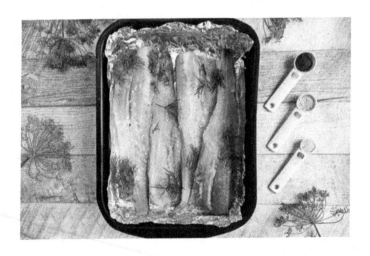

Coconut Crusted Flounder with Browned Butter and Lime

> 1/2 cup (63 g) coconut flour salt and pepper or Vege-Sal 3 eggs
> 1 1/2 pounds (680 g) flounder fillet
> 1 stick butter, divided
> 1 lime
> 4 tablespoons (16 g) minced fresh parsley

Give your big, heavy skillet a squirt of nonstick cooking spray and set it to heating over a medium burner.

On a plate, mix the coconut flour with the salt and pepper—maybe 1/4 teaspoon each.

White Clam and Bacon Pizza or Omelet Filling

4 slices bacon

1 tablespoon bacon grease (15 g) or olive oil (15 ml)

3 tablespoons (30 g) minced onion

1 teaspoon chopped garlic

1 can (6 1/2 ounces, or 180 g) minced clams

1 teaspoon Italian seasoning

1/4 cup (15 g) chopped fresh parsley

1/2 cup (58 g) 6 cheese Italian shredded cheese blend or shredded mozzarella

Lay your bacon on a microwave bacon rack or in a Pyrex pie plate and give it 4 to 6 minutes on high in the microwave.

Over medium heat, melt the bacon grease (this would be from bacon you cooked some other time—you are keeping your bacon grease to cook with, right? If you don't have bacon grease, use olive oil) in a medium-sized skillet and start sautéing the onion. While that's happening, open and drain the clams and chop your parsley.

When the onion's translucent, add the garlic, drained clams, and Italian seasoning and keep cooking until most of the residual liquid cooks away. Stir in the parsley and give it just another minute.

Okay, now you have a choice: You can make omelets according to *Dana's Easy Omelet Method*, putting 1/4 cup (30 g) of cheese in first, then the clam mixture, and topping with two strips of crumbled bacon. Or you can make tortilla pizzas, layering the same way, but heating the oven might run you past 15 minutes.

Yield: 2 servings, each with 471 calories, 29 grams fat, 43 grams protein, 9 grams carbohydrate, 1 gram dietary fiber, and 8 grams usable carb.

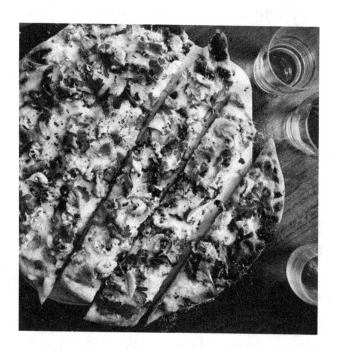

Microwaved Fish and Asparagus with Tarragon Mustard Sauce

Microwaving is a great way to cook vegetables and a great way to cook fish—so it's a natural way to cook combinations of the two.

10 asparagus spears

2 tablespoons (30 g) sour cream

1 tablespoon (14 g) mayonnaise

1/4 teaspoon dried tarragon

1/2 teaspoon Dijon or spicy brown mustard

12 ounces (340 g) fish fillets—whiting, tilapia, sole, flounder, or any other mild white fish

Snap the bottoms off the asparagus spears where they break naturally. Place the asparagus in a large glass pie plate, add 1 tablespoon (15 ml) of water, and cover by placing a plate on top. Microwave on High for 3 minutes.

While the asparagus is microwaving, stir together the sour cream, mayonnaise, tarragon, and mustard.

Remove the asparagus from the microwave, take it out of the pie plate, and set it aside. Drain the water out of the pie plate. Place the fish fillets in the pie plate and spread 2 tablespoons (28 g) of the sour cream mixture over them. Recover the pie plate and microwave the fish for 3 to 4 minutes on High. Open the microwave, remove the plate from the top of the pie plate, and arrange the asparagus on top of the fish. Recover the pie plate and cook for another 1 to 2 minutes on High.

Remove the pie plate from the microwave and take the plate off. Place the fish and asparagus on serving plates. Scrape any sauce that's cooked into the pie plate over the fish and asparagus. Top each serving with the reserved sauce and serve.

Yield: 2 servings, each with 4 grams of carbohydrates and 2 grams of fiber, for a total of 2 grams of usable carbs and 33 grams of protein.

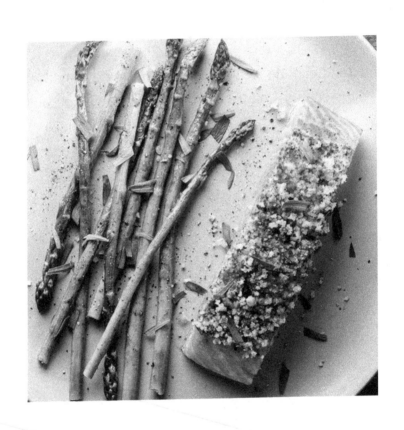

CPSIA information can be obtained
at www.ICGtesting.com
Printed in the USA
BVHW010026040521
606321BV00017B/202

9 781667 152929